Make your own e-liquid

And other tricks to make your starter kit last forever

Make your own e-liquid
Copyright © 2010 Mike Sands
ISBN: 1453873767
EAN-13: 9781453873762

Neither this entire publication nor parts of it may be reproduced, stored in or introduced into a retrieval system, or transmitted, in any form, or by any means, without having written permission from the copyright owner.

The scanning, uploading, and distribution of this book without the permission of the copyright owner is illegal and punishable by law. Please purchase only authorized electronic editions, and do not participate in or encourage electronic piracy of copyrighted materials. Your support of the author's rights is appreciated.

The author accepts no responsibility for any damage to person or property originating in experiments from this book.

The "Darwin-fish" is released into the public domain by its authors Al Seckel and John Edwards, granting anyone the right to use the work for any purpose, without conditions.

Foreword

The main purpose of this manual is to save you money! E-liquid can cost as much as a dollar for just a single milliliter, and I will teach you how to get that price down to mere pennies.

There is much talk about this on the internet but when I went to try for the first time, I found out that it was all "talk." I will take you through the entire process, including explaining in detail every step and covering all safety precautions.

In addition to this, I will also explain various methods and modifications for parts that wear out or need replacing.

Mike

Table of contents

1.	Safety equipment and precautions	5
2.	What you will need	6
3.	Making your own liquid nicotine	7
4.	Bases and liquids	9
5.	Flavorings	11
6.	Mixing	12
7.	The finished product and tweaking	14
8.	Dripping	15
9.	Atomizer modification	17
10.	Fun modifications	20
11.	Quit smoking	21
12.	Quick reference charts	22
13.	Discounts and friends	25

Chapter 1.
Safety equipment and precautions.

Nicotine in its purest form is one of the most deadly poisons known to man. With that being said, as long as the proper precautions are taken, there is no reason it cannot be handled safely.

Avoid contact with skin and eyes. If you do get it on your skin or in your eyes, flush the effected area out immediately with an abundance of clear water. It is recommended that you use rubber gloves and wear safety glasses whenever handling liquid nicotine.

Chapter 2.
What you will need.

1.5 ounce shredded tobacco.
1 measuring cup. (That measures in millimeters and ounces.)
1 small saucepan.
1 small mixing bowl.
1 handkerchief.
1 spoon.
Several small clear containers with secure lids.
1 small glass jar.
1 bottle of distilled or filtered water. (distilled is preferred)
1 bottle of vegetable glycerin. ($3 dollars at Wal-Mart)
1 bottle pure extract.
1 eyedropper.
1 ergonomical ballpoint pen.
1 pair of tweezers.
Safety glasses.
Rubber gloves.

You will need something that measures in milliliters for your mixing, and something safe and secure to hold your finished products. It will also be helpful to have a clear glass jar; you will need to see the liquid clearly to check for things like color and density. For straining, a handkerchief is preferred, but any lint free cloth will do. I once used the T-shirt I was going to wear.

To acquire something that measures in milliliters, asking your local pharmacist will probably get you what you need for free. Mine has been extremely helpful.

Chapter 3.
Making your own liquid nicotine.

Now that you have everything you need to get started, we can discuss tobacco. As with any project, you only get out of it what you put in. Taste and personal preference are everything.

You will need roughly 1.5 ounces of tobacco to get started. Hint: a normal pack of cigarettes weighs about 3/4 ounce, and so does your average size package of pipe tobacco that can be purchased for $2 at your local corner store.

You can use any tobacco you can get your hands on, but it will taste better if you use something that you personally like. You can use cigarette, cigar, pipe, or even chewing tobacco.

The first step.
Take your ground tobacco and place it into your mixing bowl. Next, fill the bowl with 3.5 cups of water. Everyone will have a different size bowl so add enough water as to where the tobacco floats in the bowl. Hint: we are going to cook out the water, so if you have a little too much it won't matter. Now you want to let it stand for 8 to 12 hours, stirring occasionally.

The second step.
After you let everything sit for 8 to 12 hours, the next thing you will want to do is separate the tobacco leaves from the water. Take the bowl and, using your cloth, strain the liquid into the saucepan. Make sure to get every drop by squeezing the water out of the leaves. Once done, discard the leaves and ring your cloth out into the saucepan, careful not to get any loose tobacco into the pan.

The third step.

Starting on a low heat, slowly bring the water to slight boil. Once it starts to boil, level out your heat and keep it at a low boil. Cooking time will vary according to the amount of liquid you have to cook down. Continue steaming away the water until nearly the entire thing has evaporated. Cook it down to anywhere between a 16th and a quarter of an inch. This may take up to an hour or more, depending on size. You want to cook it down until it becomes the consistency of syrup. Hint: it will thicken more once removed from the heat, so don't panic if your down to a 16th of an inch and yours has not thickened any yet. Once desired density is achieved, remove from heat and let cool.

Warning. At this point great care is to be taken; you now have pure nicotine and should be wearing your safety equipment.

You want your finished product to be syrupy. If it is too thick to pour or work with after cooling, simply add a little distilled or filtered water to it until it becomes a workable consistency. Do not use regular tap water due to the minerals in the water being unhealthy to vape.

When you have just the right texture, pour your mixture into a small container with a secure lid. This is now pure nicotine and should be handled with extreme care. (Image #1) No light should be seen passing through the liquid.

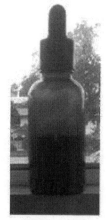

Image #1, pure nicotine. Shown in color on cover.

Chapter 4.
Bases and liquids.

There are two basic fluids used to create vapor. The first is Propylene glycol. This product has long been approved by the FDA. It is in many everyday products you already use. It is the number one ingredient in your deodorant, the number four ingredient in your toothpaste, and so on. It is also used as a food additive.

The second, and in my opinion, the better of the two, is Vegetable glycerin. Vegetable glycerin can be purchased at Wal-Mart for $3 for a 177 ml bottle. When purchasing vegetable glycerin, make sure you see the letters "USP" in the upper right hand corner. These letters mean it is safe for human consumption.

The entire purpose of this is to get the best, safest, purest, and yes, cheapest E-liquid, so for the rest of this tutorial vegetable glycerin will be used. If you personally prefer Propylene glycol, simply use it the same way you would use the vegetable glycerin.

There are two differences between the two liquids. The Propylene glycol gives a slightly better throat hit, but the vegetable glycerin produces more vapor. Warning: some people may be allergic to the Propylene glycol, which is why most reputable E-liquid dealers now offer both. Unless it is stated that vegetable glycerin is used, the odds are it is propylene glycol, or a combination of the two. The truth is, there is no sure way to know what they will send you.

Distilled water is also necessary. Both Propylene glycol and vegetable glycerin are very thick liquids and will need to be diluted a bit to achieve a workable texture.

If the liquid is too thick, you risk the chance of ruining your atomizer, which already has a limited lifespan.

If your mix is too thin, there is a risk of it running out through the bottom of your atomizer, and this can become a real problem if you're using a battery that's not sealed.

A good basic rule of thumb to go by is 15% distilled water, 15% flavoring, and 70% vegetable glycerin. This will give you a good basic E-juice, which provides tons of vapor and is easy to work with.

Chapter 5.
Flavorings.

There are a couple of different ways to add flavor to your E-liquid. There are many companies out there that sell flavorings for E-liquid. One such company is LorAnn candy oils. But don't go whipping out your credit card just yet. Extracts, sold at every grocery store will work just fine. Be careful to only buy "pure" extract. Imitation extracts contain additives that might be unhealthy to vape.

The benefit of flavor oils is that they are super concentrated. (Which will be discussed later.) For now, we are still trying to keep our costs as low as possible, so we will continue on with the extracts. Vanilla is probably the most popular E-liquid flavor out there, so go ahead and pick up a bottle, or any flavor that strikes your fancy while you're standing in the store, as long as it says it's pure.

E-liquid oils.

The one thing to keep in mind when comparing flavoring oils and extracts is that flavoring oils are 5 times more concentrated. If you choose to use these instead of extracts, what you want to do is this:

Take your unflavored E-liquid and add 25 drops of flavoring oil for every 5 milliliters of unflavored E-liquid, (vegetable glycerin, distilled water, and nicotine, as discussed in chapter 6,) and adjust to taste.

Chapter 6.
Mixing.

We are going to start by making our unflavored non-nicotine base E-liquid first. Start with your vegetable glycerin. Pour approximately 70 millimeters into your clear glass container. (Old jelly jars work great for this.)

Next, add 15 milliliters of distilled water to it. Don't worry if it's too thick at this point, you still have flavoring to add later, which will thin it out further. You should now have roughly 85 milliliters of semi thick liquid.

The next step is to add your liquid nicotine. If you took your gloves and safety glasses off, you want to put them back on now that we are handling the raw nicotine. Using your eyedropper, drip in only 8 to 10 drops of your liquid nicotine. Stir the combination of liquids together and hold it up to the light. What you want to see is a nice semi transparent caramel colored liquid. (See image #2 and 3)

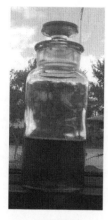

Image #2
(shown in color on cover)

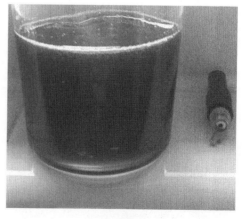

Image #3

Everyone is different. This may not be strong enough for you personally; this will be remedied in the "Tweaking" portion of this text. The nicotine you made is very strong and concentrated, so start with a very small amount, and then later add more to taste. Warning, add too much nicotine and you may make yourself ill.

Now that you have your unflavored E-juice, go ahead and add your flavoring of choice. Start by adding 15 milliliters of your flavor extract and once again stir the combination of liquids. Once your flavoring has been added and stirred in, you should have approximately 100 milliliters of E-liquid for under ten dollars.

Chapter 7.
The finished product and tweaking.

Congratulations, you now have your finished product. It should not need any tweaking at this point, and if you did everything right, it's ready to vape and enjoy. But, like I said before everyone is different. Check your finished product very carefully. Is it too thick? If so, simply add a small amount of distilled water to thin it out a bit, or if you are a flavor hound, add a little more extract.

Is it too thin and runny? Simply add a little vegetable glycerin to thicken it up a bit. Now that you have the perfect mixture there is only one thing left to do and that's to try it. Is it not strong enough for you? Just add some more of your nicotine juice. Be careful and listen to your body, only you know what is right for you. I would only add one or two drops at a time until you have the strength that is right for you.

Does it seem too strong for your tastes? Using the same 15/15/70 ratio, add some more water/flavoring/glycerin to taste. And it's just that simple; you have now made your own E-liquid personally suited to your tastes. If it's still not the flavor you are looking for, it's also possible to purchase flavor oils online which claim to taste the same as many of the popular cigarette brands.

As always, keep this and all E-liquids away from children. Even diluted Nicotine is still considered a poison.

Chapter 8.
Dripping.

Your basic E-cigarette consists of three main parts. I use, and will cover the most popular model, the Joye 510, also known as the Titan E-cig. The three parts are the battery, the atomizer, and the cartridge.

The Atomizer is the working part of the cigarette; it is what converts your E-liquid into vapor. The Cartridge is what holds the E-liquid and feeds it to the atomizer. It is recommended that this cartridge be replaced every other day, or more frequently. If you are lucky, you can buy these in bulk for 41 cents a piece. The cartridge casing is hard plastic and will theoretically last forever; it is the poly fiber inside that becomes clogged and tired.

With that being said, the first thing you can do to start saving money is to switch to the "dripping" method of vaping. A drip tip can be purchased online for anywhere from 5 to 20 dollars. What a drip tip does is allows you to drip your E-liquid directly onto the bridge of the atomizer. This is one thing that will not need to be replaced like your ordinary cartridge.

Things to consider about dripping are these: When dripping, it can be easier to flood your atomizer. I suggest to only add the amount of E-liquid that you plan on vaping at that particular moment. No more than three drops at a time is recommended. The best thing to do is: from the threaded side of the atomizer, blow through it to remove any built up juice that may be inside. Once you know you have a dry atomizer, add three drops of your E-liquid through the drip tip. Vape until dry, and repeat.

Keep that credit card in its holster still. A drip tip can easily be made at home for about 39 cents. What you need is a basic ergonomical pen. (The ones with the rubber grips on them. refer to picture #4)

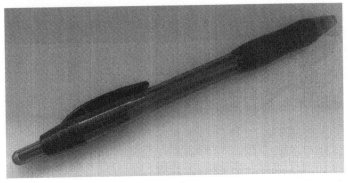

Image #4

Pull off the rubber grip and gut the pen. If you have one with the steel tip on it, simply unscrew it and set it next to the grip. If not, and you have one with a fixed plastic tip. you are going to have to cut it. (See image #5)

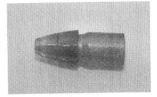

Image #5

If you don't have a coping or hack saw available, a serrated knife will work just fine. Cut your tip off at about 3/4 as long as the grip. You need the grip longer to slide over the atomizer and still hold your tip.

Slide the rubber grip over your atomizer and slide in the tip you cut off pointy side first. Now you have your own drip tip for 39 cents.

Chapter 9.
Atomizer modification.

The average life of an atomizer (according to the manufacturer) is 14 to 60 days. In reality, it is anywhere from 1 day to three months. Really, there is no way to tell how long your atomizer will last you. Don't go spending money on a new atomizer just yet though. The reason an atomizer stops producing vapor is because the steel mesh covering the bridge inside it wears out. However, this steel mesh covering the bridge of the atomizer is not needed. For that matter, neither is the bridge itself.

Odds are your atomizer still heats up, it just doesn't produce vapor any more. If this happens, don't throw it way, instead do this: Taking a pair of tweezers, reach inside the atomizer from the top (where the cartridge goes in.) Taking your tweezers, carefully move the steel mesh from the bridge of the atomizer (See image #6.)

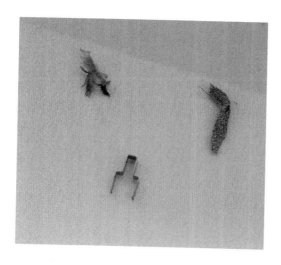

Image #6
Contents of an atomizer

Next, get a good hold of the bridge and gently yet firmly wiggle it out of the atomizer, taking care not the break the ceramic inside. Once the bridge is out, go ahead and remove the steel mesh. When you do this, you will also notice a tiny rope wick. Remove all of this loose debris, and as before blow through the atomizer from the threaded side. This will remove any remaining debris. Once this is done you should end up with a hole in the bottom of the atomizer where the bridge was. (See image #7)

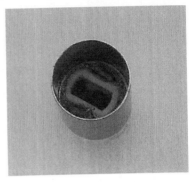

Image #7

What you don't see, however, is the fact that below the base of the atomizer is more of the steel mesh, actually more than several layers of it.

Now that your atomizer is gutted out, go ahead and once again place 3 drops of E-fluid directly down the middle of the hole. The layers of steel mesh wrapped around the heating coil inside will now be what holds your E-liquid.

This works great with a drip tip, and as with dripping, as mentioned before, be careful not to over fill and flood your atomizer.

Non drip tip method.

You don't necessarily need a drip tip to use this method. The main selling point of a drip tip is the fact that you don't need to remove the tip every time you want to top off your E-liquid. All you need is one of your old cartridges.

Make your own e-liquid

First, remove the poly fiber filling and toss it off to the side. Drip your fluid into the hole and pop your completely empty cartridge back on and vape away to your heart's content without replacing your cartridges or burned out atomizer. (See image #8.)

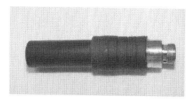

Image #8

By now, you have learned how to save money by making your own E-liquid for pennies on the dollar. You have also learned the tricks the old vapor's use to make their E-cigs a lot less "disposable". Now you don't have to throw away money replacing cartridges or atomizers!

Chapter 10.
Fun modifications.

Now that the work is done it's time to have a little fun with our E-ciggy. There are two things you can do to have fun. One mod you can try is to take another old burned out atomizer and play surgeon on it. Start by dissecting it. Remove the outer casing and atomizer bridge. Continue by removing all the metal mesh wrapped around the guts of the atomizer. Once you are this far into it, you should be able to see the two tiny wires that power the heating coil. Go ahead and snip these wires. Using any standard LED flashlight, take out the bulb, leaving some wire attached. Simply solder the bulb wires to the atomizer wires and re-assemble the atomizer. You can use 1 to 3 bulbs for this mod. You are only limited by the room inside the atomizer. And presto! Instant mini flashlight powered by your E-cig battery!

For just a couple dollars by the pharmacy at Wal-Mart you can pick up a small keychain pill holder. (They are used by heart patients for nitro tablets.) This is a perfect way to hold your flashlight mod on a keychain and keep it with you. You never know when you are going to need a flashlight. And, you know you'll have your E-cig handy to power it. It is also a handy way to carry spare atomizers.

The second mod is almost identical to the first. Only this time you solder on the inside of a laser pointer and re-assemble. This can be carried the same way on your key chain as the flashlight. The perfect mod for that up-and-coming executive inside of us all.

Chapter 11.
Quit Smoking

I have included a mixing chart for three different strength levels; low, medium, and high. If you consider yourself a heavy smoker, you are going to want to start with the "high" strength right off. Make 1 100ml bottle of each strength. That is roughly the equivalent of 30 cartons of cigarettes. By the time you get through the third bottle, "low," you find you no longer have anywhere near as strong a physical addiction to nicotine. After that, you are more than ready to go to a non nicotine E-liquid and enjoy the pleasures of pure guilt free vaping. There are literally hundreds of flavors out there for you to experiment with. Just follow this handy guide for your mixing.

The reason this works: even though you are cutting back on your nicotine intake, you are still getting the same number of puffs, and the same flavors sensations. It is this along with many other benefits that make E-cigarettes without a doubt the greatest smoking alternative known to man.

Don't panic if you are not 100% smoke free the first day! (Many people are.) The more you use your E-cigarette, the less, and less, you will be dependent on analog cigarettes. As the days go by, you will find yourself smoking fewer and fewer analogs. Remember, it's not always about how many analog cigarettes you smoke, it's about how many you are able to avoid smoking!

Chapter 12.
Quick reference charts.

Mixing
15% Flavorings
15% Distilled water
70% Vegtable glycerin.

25 drops of flavor oils for every 5 milliliters unflavored E-liquid.

Strengths
Low   5 drops of liquid nicotine per 100 ml base
Medium   10 drops of liquid nicotine per 100 ml base
High   15 drops of liquid nicotine per 100 ml base

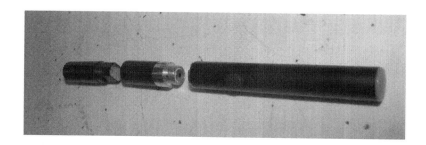

510-series e-cigarette. From left to right above are the Cartridge, the Atomizer, and the Battery. This is a manual battery with a button to press when vaping, there are also automatic batteries that turn on when you use them. To the far right is the diode that glows when vaping, giving a sense of a "real" cigarette.

Below is the 510 put together, looking much like an analog cigarette. The parts come in many different colors.

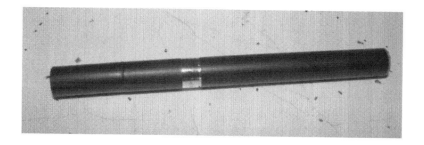

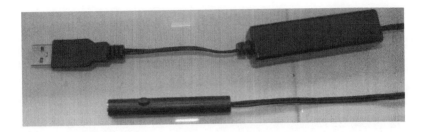

The picture above shows a pass-through. This allows you to vape connected to a computer, or to the power-outlet through an adapter. There is a replaceable battery in the black box to the upper right. **Warning**: the batteries look like standard AAA but they are not. Be careful to check the voltage when replacing!

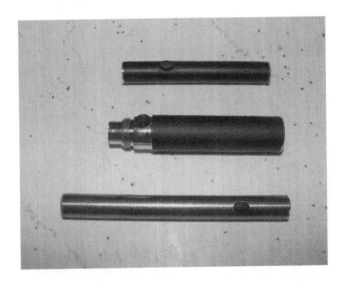

E-cigarettes come in many shapes and sizes. Above are three different kinds of batteries that all work with the 510 atomizers and cartridges. Bigger batteries last longer, and take longer to charge.

Chapter 13.
Discounts and friends.

By now, you can make your starter kit last indefinitely, but you still need to get that starter kit from somewhere. So far the best value for the money comes from http://www.totallywicked-eliquid.com The 510 series, which has been used for this tutorial, is only $29.99 at the time of writing the book, plus shipping, with no strings attached. With this kit, you will receive 1 x Manual Battery, 1 x Atomizer, 1 x USB Charger, 1 x 10ml Bottle of 18mg Tobacco or Menthol E-Liquid, and 3 x 510 refillable Cartridges.

Still going with the "save you money," there is also a coupon code to get an additional 7.5% off of the $29.99 price. The code is dcf9d. This code is good for anything they sell that's not already discounted, and will never expire.

Flavorings can be purchased directly from the manufacturer at https://www.lorannoils.com

If you find yourself still unsure about making your own E-liquid the best place out there to buy some (great prices and incredible customer service) is http://cleancigs.com You can get your choice from non-nicotine all the way up to super high 36mg strength. You can also specify what type of base you want from PG to VG to a mixture of the two.

Lastly, and quite possibly the most important. If you are looking for a good read to vape, do yourself a favor and look up Maria Hammarblad at http://www.amazon.com A great author and the inspiration for me to switch from analogs to E-cigs.

Starter kits.
http://www.totallywicked-eliquid.com
Use coupon code DCF9D

Flavor oils.
https://www.lorannoils.com

E-liquid.
http://cleancigs.com

Vape read.
http://www.amazon.com/maria_hammarblad

Made in the USA
Lexington, KY
15 April 2013